Get Real With
RECOVERY

Get Real With
RECOVERY

Darnel Dickerson

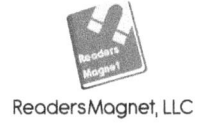

ReadersMagnet, LLC

Get Real With Recovery
Copyright © 2020 by Darnel Dickerson

Published in the United States of America
ISBN Paperback: 978-1-951775-65-0
ISBN eBook: 978-1-951775-66-7

All rights reserved. No part of this publication may be reproduced, stored in a retrieval system or transmitted in any way by any means, electronic, mechanical, photocopy, recording or otherwise without the prior permission of the author except as provided by USA copyright law.

The opinions expressed by the author are not necessarily those of ReadersMagnet, LLC.

ReadersMagnet, LLC
10620 Treena Street, Suite 230 | San Diego, California, 92131 USA
1.619.354.2643 | www.readersmagnet.com

Book design copyright © 2020 by ReadersMagnet, LLC. All rights reserved.
Cover design by Ericka Obando
Interior design by Shemaryl Tampus

If you learn nothing from your mistakes in life, you stop growing… Don't refuse to learn.

It takes just as long to see the good things in life as it does to see the bad. Make sure you dedicate time to focus on the good and not dwell on the bad.

Contents

Foreword	9
Special Thanks To	11
The Solution	23
Where Do We Start?	24
Dare To Dream, Dare To Live That Dream	49
Relationship And Recovery	51
Other Not-So-Good Things About Addiction	55

FOREWORD

Do you remember the dreams you dreamed as a kid? We all had dreams, like being a movie star or fireman, or football player... We dreamed good dreams and envisioned prosperous things.

As a child, I was a big dreamer. I dreamed of being rich like other members of my family, by means of owning my own business, or being the leader of a large company. In those dreams I was very rich and I helped others. The dream I envisioned carried me from high school to college and also to the military. I needed and wanted skills. The dream to be successful is what kept me going.

My dream, I could picture it clear as day: me leaving my huge home to go work in one of my companies, driving a very nice and expensive car. With all the people answering to me. Nice dream, yeah?

Not once in any of my recalled memories do I remember dreaming of becoming a full-time drug user, jailbird, family disgrace, thief, child abuser (mentally, not physically), and menace to society.

There are several things and events that alter some people's dreams. Some of us alter our hopes and dreams on our own! In my opinion, this is a tragic thing we do to ourselves.

Get Real with Recovery brings hope and ideas so you can live sober and achieve a path to your dreams.

SPECIAL THANKS TO

The counselor Charles Moose at Parallax in Wichita, Kansas, for advising me on a solid recovery plan. Tony B., my sponsor who helped me over some very rough humps. Thank you for your dedication to the recovery program.

My wife, who hung in through the worst nightmares any one person should never have to endure. Yet you saw in me what I couldn't even see in myself at that time. Thank you, I love you forever and a day.

My family: the support you showed me every day and the non-enabling you did helped me detour my addiction. I apologize for any embar-rassment and misrepresentation I caused our family. Thank you for not turning your backs or losing hope that God could and would return me to sanity.

Thank you to my editor for showing patience and helping me with this project. I couldn't have gotten it right without you.

Extra special thanks to God Almighty, for without you there is no me.

I will start this book by saying, first and foremost, thank you for taking interest in recovery for yourself, and for choosing my book as an additional tool to help you achieve your goal.

In this book I use a lot of my past experiences as reference to the addict. I am an addict! But I am an addict who is in recovery. Many of the promises of recovery have come true for me. I am so happy about my life and what seems to be a new meaning to my life. I want to share with those who are still suffering, what happened back then and what's happening now.

The reason I want to do this is with hope that those who read Get Real with Recovery will see that if I can do it, anyone can. It is also with hope that my story and the real facts will inspire many to want to strive for the real recovery.

I'm not talking the hit-and-miss recovery where you try, but the real recovery where you do it.

My name is Darnel Dickerson. I was a good kid growing up. I came from a good home. My mother raised me and my three sisters on her own. Yet and still, she taught us all the reality of life and respect that was to be shown at all times. I was a good student in school and learned the work ethic at an early age. I grew up like the average kid with siblings. We did our share of arguing, fussing, and fighting. In our home there were no drugs or alcohol. Like with almost all families, there was some sort of dysfunction, but none that should have led me to the life of using drugs.

Where did it all begin? I started smoking pot when I was thirteen years old. It was a casual thing at first. Smoking after school and weekends with my neighborhood buddies. By the time I was graduating high school, I was smoking anytime I could. I would do things like wake up in the morning and smoke weed (wake-n-bake). I would ditch some of my high school classes to go get high. I would smoke weed on the way to work and while I was working. Yes, I was a full-time pothead at an early age.

Ironically, I had no major or noticeable, significant consequences due to my pot smoking. My grades were good all the way through school. (My mother would not have had it any other way.) I was never in trouble with the law. (She wasn't going to tolerate that, either.)

My consequences began more when I graduated to the narcotic, cocaine. Don't get this twisted; I'm not saying that smoking weed had no consequences. They just were nowhere near the magnitude of trouble that consumed my life once I started using cocaine.

I tend to take a look back in the rearview mirror because I never want to forget where I came from. I figured, as should you, that if I closed the door on my past and tried to forget what happened, I would have learned nothing from the experience.

As you read, I urge you to write about or draw your own Positive Thoughts and Ideas, Looking Forward Dreams, To-Do List, Amends List, Promises, Personal Goals, and Achievements on the pages at the back of the book. This is a tool you can use to your benefit. You might want to place dates on the pages to track your progress.

No matter how bad it was, we still need to remember the good, the bad, and the ugly. These things were all lessons.

We may have had some hard, costly, and maybe even very embarrassing lessons, yet and still they are all lessons.

I feel that if you can learn from your past experiences, they can propel you forward in your future to know what not to do. This is called wisdom. We all need to be wiser. Don't you agree?

By looking back, you see the things you have done that may have hurt you and others while you were in your addiction. If indeed you are serious about getting recovery, you will want to keep in mind the insane behavior that got you on a downhill spiral. It is my belief that by looking back, you will keep the path clear from making the same dreaded and insane mistakes you constantly made while using.

I remember failing myself over and over again. My recovery program was not a solid one.

I had recovery by jail. It didn't work.

Recovery by force. Court-ordered treatment. It didn't work either.

There was recovery by finance, which occurred only after I had spent all my money, hawked all my valuables, and took as much as I could from others without seemingly being noticed (stealing).

Then comes the recovery by guilt. Feeling guilty about all of the above and knowing this was not the way you were raised or the way you want to live… feeling guilty for not being the responsible person you know you can be or ought to be.

You see, all of these are forms of recovery, however none of those forms of recovery work!

Here is where the reality of recovery begins to set in. If you for one minute think you can do this without any help… if you think you can quit on your own… you are going to relapse—and in a bad way.

There is no soft or easy way to get recovery. Very few are successful at quitting using drugs without any help. If you think this may be you... I wish you good luck.

Being realistic, you cannot quit without help! Let me break it down for you. Your best thinking got you stuck on drugs. And even if you have not been a career drug user, if you have used more than once, you have a problem.

In getting clean there are many variables, and many tools to help you stay clean. When I say clean, I mean a clean lifestyle. Clean lifestyle and recovery are one and the same. However, recovery and clean are two different things.

Being clean (clean time) only means the length of time that you have not used. We accomplish clean time when we are put in jail. This does not mean we are in recovery. We get clean time when our money runs out. This is not recovery either! I'm sure you get the point.

Recovery comes when you make the conscious decision to not use drugs or alcohol, and to move forward with your life. I have found that most people relapse because they only got clean; they had not begun their recovery.

There is a difference. When you are clean, the only thing you have done is not used. Your same old behavior is there. You have done nothing to prepare yourself for long-term sobriety. You simply are not getting high.

With recovery, you are not only not using, but are also taking steps necessary to stay not using. You need the tools and knowledge to keep you from using. Not just trying to stop. You want to stay stopped? You need to know how. Or it won't last long... Your not using, that is.

In getting clean and sober and moving towards true recovery from your addiction, you only have to change one thing. And the one thing you have to change is EVERYTHING!

The people who actually get recovery and keep it are the ones who changed that one thing. You can't honestly expect to get and keep your recovery and still do the same things as you have always done. If you do, again, you are sadly mistaken.

For example, you can't expect to go hang out with the people you used with and not want to use too, if you see them using or if they have used.

Face this realistically. Can you put an alcoholic in a bar and expect him not to drink? I think you already know that's not gonna work. So it works the same way with your using. You cannot go places where you used to. You cannot hang out with people you have used with, and it's certainly not good to hang out in an environment where the temptation to use is there. Chances are you will use.

You have to build a new routine. Some of the biggest triggers that lead to using are the things that you normally do. That's part of why you have to change everything.

For some of us, this is a very tough thing to do. Apart from building a new routine, you have to leave Pookie, Junebug, and Ray Ray alone. When I say Pookie, Junebug, and Ray Ray, you put your using friends' names there instead.

The hard part about this is… some of our using friends, we actually like or care about. Sometimes those Pookies, Junebugs, and Ray Rays are family members. It can be very difficult to let go of these people.

You have to make a choice. This is a dog-eat-dog world. It would seem to be a no-brainer, and recovery is more important. Some of our using friends are old friends and family. But which would you rather have, your same old friends, same consequences, same life as you know it now?

Or would you rather have the life you and your family truly deserve? Even if you are not married or don't have children, you still may have other family members. Let's face it, we represent our families, good, bad, or indifferent. We do. Even if you have no family, you owe it to yourself to live better than what drugs and alcohol allow.

Do you really think you can carry on a meaningful relationship with another person while immersed in an addiction? What about a true friendship?

Let's talk about the relationship first. I say from experience, the quality of a meaningful relationship starves. The impact that cocaine, meth, heroin, and alcohol have on the individual are not a positive one. So, in reality, how can anything positive come from something that's negative?

Now let's talk about friendships. Can you truly trust the people you use with?

Let me ask this:

- When you were using, did you ever leave your dope or your money laying around?

- Did you ever lend money to someone else you knew was using?

- If you did, did you get it back?

- And if you did get it back, how long did it take to get it back?

Let's hope you answered these questions honestly, and you see my point.

You cannot have a quality anything when on drugs. We as addicts have to quit taking the Road to Nowhere and move on to better things.

Not to mention what we sacrifice to go get high. Leaving our responsibilities to tend to themselves, our family's confidence in us tends to waver.

Realistically, many of us have tried, and maybe even succeeded to a degree, to quit using on our own and maintain a meaningful relationship with our friends and family.

If we are honest with ourselves, we as addicts leave a lot to be desired in the relationship department. At least at a good quality level.

To better your chances of recovery, as hard as it may seem, you must distance yourself from those using friends and associates—even if they are family.

If any of them are good friends, they will respect your decision to get clean and try a different way of life. If these "friends" care about you any, they will support your efforts, and not hinder you in your decision to try recovery. Again, if they care, they will even distance themselves from you.

Keep in mind the old adage that "Misery loves company." No one wants to be miserable by themselves. So, more than likely, Pookie, Junebug, and Ray Ray will disregard your efforts and try to get you to keep doing what you have been with them.

Think about this, because you contributed to their high, too. Be it your money, your connection, your hustle, whatever it was you did to bring your share of the drugs you used together to the table. If you are not there with them, that's less dope for them, and it's scary for them, as it is for you, to get recovery. It may take a while for them to find a replacement for your share or what you contributed. Don't get it twisted; they will find a replacement.

Think again from another perspective: What happened when you went to jail? This may not have happened to you. You may never have had that consequence of being arrested. But the reality is most of us as addicts have been put in jail for something. Maybe for not paying a ticket or not showing up for court. These may be indirect reasons, but most of the indirect reasons also lead back to using and not taking care of our responsibilities. Anyway, when you were in jail, who did you call? Was it Pookie, Junebug, and Ray Ray? Did they come get you?

If you answered yes to the second question, you are among a very rare crowd of using friends. Because most using friends don't have the money to bail you out of jail. They already spent their money on drugs. And if they do bond you out, that's going to cut into their dope money.

So, what this is summing up to is, if you go to jail, those "friends" are not coming for you. But they will tell everyone else in the drug community you are in jail.

The dope community has a way of getting the word out as to what's up with each other. Who's in jail, who got busted, who got killed and why. Who died and how. It never really is good news. Isn't that

depressing? I didn't think it at the time when I was out there too. But that's because I was a part of that depressing life.

The bottom line is you cannot run around with Pookie, Junebug, and Ray Ray. It won't help you get clean.

You have to step outside your normal, everyday box! What I mean is you have to continue to make positive changes in all areas of your life.

Since I've spent time here telling you that you can't hang with using friends and family, I'll say this: Anybody who is not a part of the solution of your getting clean, they are a part of the problem of your addiction.

Take a break and doddle or write your thoughts.

Take a break and doddle or write your thoughts.

Take a break and doddle or write your thoughts.

THE SOLUTION

THERE ARE COUNTLESS WAYS TO get clean, and by no means am I saying that I have the answers for everyone's addiction. The fact is everybody's recovery is different. What I am saying is there are tested, tried and true tools to get clean and sober. But unless you are ready and really truly want to get clean and get recovery, it is useless, and any solutions offered will be a waste of your time and the time will also be wasted of those trying to help.

WHERE DO WE START?

- First you have to make a serious, conscious decision to give up the life of drugs and all the bad that comes with it. I've seen where there are those who are not only addicted to drugs, but also have an addiction to the drama that comes with them. At times, this can be worse than the addiction to drugs.

- Then you have to find a treatment facility. Whether it's inpatient or outpatient, that's going to depend on your assessment. I suggest you find a treatment center and check into detox. Be honest about your use. If you are seeking help, they will offer the help. If you don't have insurance, don't worry about it. Most of us tricked off any good jobs that may have had insurance anyway. The treatment centers often will help you find funding, if not a court order from a judge. Society sees us addicts as a menace or cancer to our society, so believe me, we want everyone to get clean and share the message of getting clean. Getting into treatment is a very important part of recovery. In treatment you learn what your triggers are and how to combat them when they arise. If you don't think you need treatment, you are in denial and more than likely will fail at recovery and will relapse. You have to know what triggers you to go use when you know you shouldn't. And in treatment you almost always find things that trigger you that you may have never thought of otherwise. I strongly urge you to take this step.

- Get a sponsor and support network. Find a good one, not somebody you can piss on and tell him it rained. Find a sharp sponsor, somebody who has been there and done that. This person should understand the life that you are leading, where you've been, and where you are trying to go. Don't be afraid of telling him or her your dark and dirty secrets. Call your sponsor regularly and do what your sponsor suggests you do.

I met my sponsor at a meeting, which is where you will probably find yours, too. He was speaking to the whole group but the things he was saying to the group, it felt like he was speaking directly to me. I related to what he was saying and I knew he'd be real with me about mine, so after that meeting I talked with him and asked if he would consider being my sponsor.

I did whatever he suggested to me. I listened because he had been where I was at, and I wanted to be where he was. I was lucky. Some people have to try many different sponsors till they find the right one. But the fact that they will keep looking if they have to is very good. They refuse to give up on themselves just because they didn't get the right sponsor the first time.

- Continue by going to CA, NA, or AA meetings on a regular basis. In meetings we meet people who share the same interests of staying clean and sober, and restoring order to their lives.

  I have found some very good friendships and support in meeting rooms of recovery.

- Your support network will probably be some of these people, but not limited to the people you encounter at meetings. I say this because they are trying to stay clean too, and will be there to listen when you are having tough moments.

  Other support you may have are non-using friends and family, like maybe your parents or grandparents, or the pastor from your church. Please, I urge you not to try counting on your old using friends for support unless they are in recovery and, hopefully, have more recovery time than you.

  What you may hear at a meeting from others who are there sharing, may turn on a light that may forever keep you clean and in recovery. It may be a story, a sentence, a phrase, or just the way someone who was just like you carries themselves, that makes the difference. Keep going to meetings, keep your sponsor and support network. It will make a difference.

- Seek a higher power. My higher power, which I choose to call God, saw me through the worst of my addiction, and now some of the best of my recovery. I strongly feel that the best is yet to come. I meditate in the mornings, I praise him during my day, and I pray at night, thanking him for bringing me through my days, and through my trials and tribulations.

I understand that not everyone believes in the same higher power. Higher power, simply put, is a power greater than self. Your higher power can be two or more people, a meeting, or whatever is bigger and stronger than you.

Here's a scenario that may help you to understand where I am coming from. If I were standing alone and someone pushed me, I might stumble or even fall. But if I have one or two people from my support network holding me and the same person pushed me, it is highly doubtful that I can be pushed around. This support is a power greater than self. This is one of many analogies to help you see that you stand a better chance with help, rather than trying to go at recovery alone.

- Another suggestion I have is one that works for me and will, without any doubt in my mind, work for anybody in recovery, or even if they have been sober their whole life.

It's a planner! As soon as possible, you buy yourself a planner and begin writing down your goals. Start with daily, spread to weekly, then monthly, and so on. By writing down your goals, you commit yourself to your goals. If you don't try achieving your goals, you only are letting yourself down.

But as you write them down, and at the end of the day you check off all the things you've accomplished, it gives you a sense of satisfaction. It also helps you organize and get lots more done than you can imagine.

Only 4 percent of people in the world write down their goals, and of that 4 percent, 100 percent of them are successful. I'm not saying they are all rich—though most of them are. I'm saying they are successful.

I'll give an example. Have you ever gone to the grocery store to buy items that you need for the home? When you get back home you realize you forgot some of the stuff you needed.

Think about when you write out a grocery list and take it with you to the store. You don't forget any of the stuff you need because you wrote out a list. The list was your goal you needed to achieve from the store.

Now relate this to your everyday life by writing down your goals. Soon you will be getting lots done and being successful while you are at it. Keep your list filled with positive things to accomplish, and what you can't get done on one day, put it on the next day's goal list.

It is my opinion that unless you put on your goal list "Get high" or "Call Pookie, Junebug, Ray Ray, or the dope man," you won't have time to get high. This will surely help you a long way in your recovery.

The dictionary defines "recovery" as "returning to an original state." Originally we were not born dope addicts. The question is… Is the original state where you want to be? You may, like I did, want something better than the original state you were in. Coming from the state of addiction, you may want to surpass your original state and move on to better than an original state of things. This is my hope for everyone seeking recovery.

Let's go back and take a look at a few things said. I reiterate these items to stress some really important methods that not only worked for me but for others as well

To really get and keep your recovery you have to change that one thing I talked about earlier. That thing is EVERYTHING. The people who seek this change are usually very successful at keeping their recovery.

You have to attend meetings. This is where you develop new friendships with people you have things in common with, who can relate to what's happening in your life. This can also help with the distance you need to put between yourself and Pookie, Junebug, and Ray Ray.

Meeting rooms are also like a safe haven; the time spent there will assist in deterring you from wanting to use. The time spent there will keep you from worrying about using and being influenced by "You Know Who" to come with them to get high. Getting clean and staying that way is one of those things you have to change.

Nothing that's worth having is easy. If it were, everyone would have it. Recovery in the beginning is not easy. It gets easier as you continue to work it. Changing everything is not easy. But just ask anyone who is living the recovery lifestyle. It is very worth it!

Here are some real questions for you. I hope you answer these questions honestly. Write your answers in the book if you want.

Without real honesty for yourself and for others, you are not going to be successful at recovery. At least not for very long. If you can't be honest to yourself, you ultimately cannot be honest with anyone else. Here are those real questions:

- Do you think you have a drug problem?

- Do you think your drug use has had any effect on any of your family members?

- Do you have a job? If not, why not?

- Do you think you can stop using anytime you want?

- Do you think you can quit on your own?

- Do you have children? Would you want your children to use drugs?

- Are you a manipulator to benefit your using?

- Do you have a conscience?

- Do you feel regret or remorse?

- Do you want a better life than what you have?

- What are you currently doing to improve your life?

- Have you hurt your health due to your use?

- Have you rotted out your teeth, or made them worse due to your use?

- Do you want to quit using?

- Do you care if you live or die?

- Do you want help to stop using?

- Where do you see yourself in two to three years?

- What are you going to do to accomplish your two- to three-year goal?

- Do you care about anything? If so, what?

It is my hope that you answered the questions honestly. They were questions asked of me, too. When you answer such questions, they make you think and process some of your life. They are not questions designed for the weak minded. They are questions to make you realize where you are at. And nudge you to act up, do something. You know… take action.

Some may still be asking exactly where they should start. Again I will reiterate that everybody is different. What may work for one may not work for another. I offer several suggestions throughout this book.

I can tell you exactly where I started. I started from what seemed to be a hopeless state of existence. I went to treatment and I listened and got the facts about recovery. I made the conscious decision that I wanted a better life. I got very honest I) with myself and I asked God for help. I found my sponsor and I did exactly what he told me. Nothing else that I had come up with had worked, so I did. what he told me because the only options I had left were a very long prison stay or death, neither of which I wanted.

My higher power (God) became for me a twenty-four-hour vigil. I prayed before my feet hit the floor every morning. I praised him throughout the day. And I thanked him every evening before going to sleep. I found that if you follow God's plan and obey God's law, you are less likely to break man's law.

I changed the company I kept. No more Pookie, Junebug, and Ray Ray. I even stayed away from family that I knew used.

I got myself a planner and started filling it up. I started making plans to make the effort to realize my dreams.

I reported to my probation officer, ready to submit a UA to him. I did lots of community service—some of which was required by my probation officer. But I went ten times or more beyond what he wanted for me. This helped keep me from having idle time.

I began to do things with my wife and kids. Besides working and going to meetings and community service, my family were the only people I was around.

This is what helped me in the start of my recovery. Again, this same plan may not work for you. You can take bits and pieces of what I did, or what someone else did, and work them into your own recovery. I promise you will see some of your dreams realized if you start working recovery first, and go after your dreams. Without recovery you won't realize anything but misery. You will not get to see any of your dreams come true.

I often feel that non-using parents, grandparents, or spouses of users should also take something like a class or read a book about recovery.

So many times I see parents and spouses enable their children or spouse. And this just keeps the user using.

Parents think they are helping their child by giving them shelter, bailing them out of jail or other jams. Giving them money, paying their delinquent bills, this helps users stay sick! You may think that you do this because you love your child and you don't want to see him or her suffer. **To love your child or spouse is commendable. But when you enable them, you are in fact making their situation worse.**

You say you love them, but you give them money for drugs. Maybe that's not what you intentionally gave them the money for. You know they have a problem. What do you think they are doing with money you give them?

You bail them out of jail and other jams because you love them. What you are actually doing is denying them their bottom. Some addicts have to reach a bottom in order to move up. You as a parent or spouse are helping to prevent them from reaching their bottom. And you are keeping them lost.

Tough love is what the addict needs. If you really love or want to help them, cut off any cash in hand to them. Don't lend them your car or buy gas for theirs. For an addict, gas in their car is a way for them to ride around to find themselves a high. They even trade their cars for a day or two of dope. They actually loan their car to their dealer in exchange for drugs.

You pay their bills and you free up pressure on them so they can concentrate on getting more drugs.

As parents, you hate to think of your child being that way… using you to keep their addiction going, but the drug has no conscience.

If you truly do want to help, then quit holding their hands, cleaning up their messes, and bailing them out of situations. Who are you to deny them their bottom? You yourself need to stop your own denial. The fact is you have a child who is an addict. If you want to help, show tough love, make them earn everything they get from you. Stop being an enabler.

Help them when you see they are helping themselves. Don't be too eager to help, either. Because they are addicts, do not doubt that they will pee on you and tell you it's rain. So don't be a softy; question everything. Even the answers they give you to your questions. Don't let them try to make you feel guilty for asking. They made the bed, let them lie in it. **Trust is to be earned, not given.**

Remember, parents, anybody can clean up for thirty days or so. Real recovery will show in ALL their actions. Who they run with, their sleeping and eating habits, their hygiene, their attitudes—and it will take longer than thirty days. So don't be a fool to the addict.

Mom/Dad, if you are not a part of the solution, you are part of the problem. A lot of time you are a part of the problem and don't even know it. Pay attention, don't allow yourself to be an enabler. You won't be helping the one you love, you'll be hurting them.

Looking back is a very big part of moving forward. If you forget where you came from, how are you gonna know if you are moving forward? You don't want to close the door or try to forget, because in that case you have learned nothing from your experience.

Don't look at your past as a crushing blow of defeat. Always use it as a steppingstone to greater accomplishments.

Just as looking back is important, in contrast, looking forward is important. Looking forward is nothing much more than planning your future: the things you want to do, need to do, or want to do. Some people call these things Looking Forward Dreams. Successful people call them Goals.

Dreams, promises, and goals. However you perceive them, look forward. I urge you to look forward to a better life. That's exactly what you are gonna get, working the steps of recovery with a support network and sponsor.

Keep in mind Pookie, Junebug, and Ray Ray are what's called fair-weather friends. They are there when you have something to offer or when you are needed for something… but so hard to find when you are in need. And when they can be found, they can't help you.

Do you remember when you were younger and your friends would come over to see if you could play? They didn't want or need anything from you; they just wanted your company.

This you will find again in recovery. Not just in recovery rooms but in recovery in general. As your self-esteem flourishes you will begin doing things that bring a sense of pride to yourself. Others will want to share in that newfound pride you carry. They will also have their own pride to bring to the table. You will have real relationships with folks who don't care only if you have money or drugs. It will be all about your character all over again. This too is a beautiful thing. I implore you to try recovery. It's great.

It's not like when you were in your addiction, and your so-called friends would want to hook up with you. They wanted to know what you had, if you could get anything, or they needed you to make a connection for them.

Friends are for support. They lift you up, they encourage, show concern, and are there when you need them. And to have a friend, you must first be a friend.

By no means does a real friend encourage his friend to use. A real friend helps you succeed, and does not hinder your success by helping you stay stuck like they are. And by your trying to be a good friend and wanting to get clean, ask your friend to join you in getting help, to get clean. If they go along with you, great. If not, distance yourself til you have a handle on recovery. Then they may want what you have, and you can show them the path you took.

You can't wait for them or expect them to just follow you. Those are things that happen in addiction. You can lead by example and hope they will want what you have.

Someone who is not your friend will try to tell you how you can get high and what to use to clear your system when they know you are trying to quit or would have legal consequences if you did use.

They don't have to live your life and don't care how it turns out. Remember, they don't have to do your time if you go to jail, nor do they have to walk in your shoes. As I said before, misery loves company.

It's not easy to decipher who these friends are at first. The longer you keep clean and not use, and follow a plan for recovery, you will begin more and more to figure out who is there to help. Again, if they are not a part of the solution, they are definitely part of the problem.

Recovery is a selfish program where you have to get into yourself to figure yourself out and what triggers you to use. No matter how selfish this program of recovery is, you can't do it alone.

We all know that not using is a step up from using. Not to say those in recovery are any better than those who are still in their addiction, we are just better off. We have greater opportunities.

Let's be real. We don't qualify for decent jobs when we are in an addiction, nor is our health as good. Also consider the money saved by not giving it to our dope dealer.

The trust in yourself grows, and trust is earned back from those who lost trust in us because of our addiction.

Trust is to be earned, not given. So don't be mad when you get into recovery and those you hurt while in your addiction don't immediately trust you. You may have done a lot of damage to them, maybe irreparable damage.

Just like your addiction showed in time, so will your recovery. It will show. If you are truly in recovery, it will show in you.

It will show in your attitude.

It will show in job stability.

It will show in your integrity.

It will show in all you do.

It may take time, but it will show. This is a fact. In true recovery you will try to make amends to those you hurt. It may not happen right away, but it will happen for the most part.

Be involved with your recovery, participate in the meetings you go to. Offer to do service work. As your strength comes back to you... you will meet others who need your help.

I know you can do great things in your life. I believe we all have the capacity to live clean and sober. Be bold, take a chance on yourself. You'll discover your best hasn't passed you, it (your best) is yet to come.

Your support network: Use them not only for the bad times you have while focusing on recovery, but also use them on your good days.

I have had people tell me that they think they could do this program of recovery alone. I don't think it impossible. Those who try this... I wish them luck. But your best thinking has made you an addict. So good luck with that. For the most part, these people relapse and their chances are way less than those who seek help. Why chance it? If you want it, you have to learn it.

There are so many people in recovery that I guarantee will help you if you ask. That's part of their recovery, too. In order to keep recovery, you have to give it away. Whatever you learn for yourself from this program is priceless, yet and still, you have to give it to another who needs it. **If your addiction has made you feel useless, your recovery will show you that you are useful in more ways than one.**

You will find people, having from just a couple of months to many years of clean time, who are willing to help others with recovery. It's how they stay grounded and maintain their recovery.

Don't for one minute think you can go to a treatment class and get through it, that then you are cured. There is no cure. **You have to maintain recovery.** It's like working on your car. Because you took it to the shop or fixed it yourself doesn't mean you are never going to have problems with it again. You know as well as I do if you don't keep your car maintained, it's gonna break down.

Same thing goes for your recovery. If you don't keep it tuned up, it's gonna break down too. Keep in touch with your sponsor, keep going to meetings to keep yourself tuned up. It also helps the newcomer and that's a load of encouragement to those who don't know if they can do it. **Remember, if I can, you can.** And that rubs off on others. It can go from me to you, and from you to someone else, so on and so forth.

You can save someone's life with your recovery. That's a meaningful thing to do with your life. I'm always willing to help with the recovery of another, as will you when you begin to grasp recovery of your own.

Let's move forward, not backwards. I have heard people say that relapse is a part of recovery—that you have to fall off the proverbial bike to learn how to ride.

I ask you this: When you took your first driving lessons, did you wreck the car you were learning in? Or did you get a little nervous and maybe hit the gas pedal too hard or brake too hard, and then your driving instructor advised you what to do to become a smooth driver?

That's how I view recovery. You may not know it very well, but there are those who could teach it to you. Just like your driving instructor taught you to drive. A sponsor, a counselor, or support network can guide you on how to smooth out some of the rough spots in recovery.

You don't wake up one day and say "I'm not using anymore." Although I've heard it happens, but not very often.

Let's get real. How long did you get high? Now, are you prepared to spend at least that same amount of time working on recovery? If you do spend that much time working on recovery, you will be amazed at all you accomplish to the good, in half the time of your addiction.

Take a break and doodle or write your thoughts here or in the back of the book.

I have shared some facts and some opinions with you. There are so many more facts that you can obtain and so many sources to get these facts.

There is the Alcoholics Anonymous Big Book, which was lent to the Cocaine Anonymous name. It is followed because it has been proven to work.

The Twelve Steps and Twelve Traditions are derived from the AA Book. There is a ton of literature for the drug you choose to lose. If you hunt for this literature the way you hunted for the drug of your choice, I guarantee you will find it.

I know from experience that most addicts are pretty smart. I'm not saying we all have superior IQs or anything like that. What I'm saying is, to a certain degree, we have the ability to know what's right and what's wrong. When we or most of us started using, we knew what we were doing was wrong and even illegal. But we did it anyway. To party with our friends or maybe to fit in with our peers, for this we made poor judgments. As our addiction progressed, we made further poor and irrational decisions.

These decisions and poor judgments not only affect us, but also our families and society as a whole. We tell ourselves that we aren't hurting anybody but ourselves. And the thing is, we tell ourselves that and we know it is a boldfaced lie.

Here is a series of questions that I am going to ask. Answer them to yourself but do so honestly. Don't lie to yourself.

Think real hard about who your best friend is. Picture how strongly you feel about this person, the one you trust and love the most.

Now answer these questions.

• What would you do if your best friend took your money out of your wallet?

• What would you do if you confronted your best friend and he/she hit you over the head with a tire iron, called the police, told the police you took his money and hit him/her with the tire iron?

• What would you do if, when you got your one phone call from jail, your best friend answered your phone and told you he/she was sleeping with your wife/husband?

...About now, I'm wondering what your answers are. But I'm not finished with my questions.

• What would you do if you found out your best friend moved into your house while you were sitting in jail?

• What would you do if you found out your best friend was slapping your kids around?

So, let's recap to make sure you have this right. Your best friend took your money, hit you over the head, put you in jail, he/she is answering your phone, sleeping with your wife/husband, moved into your house, and is slapping your kids around.

What would you do? If you answered with anything less than, you would embrace your best friend fondly, and telling him/her that's it's all good, you need to check yourself for honesty.

As an addict, your best friend is the drug you use. And by that drug being your best friend, it has done all those things and maybe more to you. Yet you always seem to run back to that friend and embrace that friend, to continue to treat you like that.

Is this rational behavior? Looking at it from this perspective, it seems so insane. That is exactly my point. We are not stupid people. The drugs we use make us do stupid things we would otherwise not do.

We have to distance ourselves from using and those using friends so we don't have to make what appear to be stupid decisions.

You are a leader by not knowing who you are. I say you are a leader because much of the world population is comprised of natural-born leaders. They just have not developed those leadership skills and some never know they have them. But in order to lead, you must first follow. Thus I stress to you the importance of a sponsor. My sponsor, Tony B., has been the only sponsor I've ever had and I still call him to this very day.

We are friends and discuss many topics, not just the topic of recovery. I chose my sponsor because I knew I couldn't walk over him. I knew he would call me on my stuff and question me to make sure I stayed straight up.

Tony B. has inspired me and guided me so far for about four years. This is a real friend now, despite the fact I barely knew him when he became my sponsor.

The point I'm trying to make here is that I now have a friend in recovery. It's a quality friendship not found in an addiction situation. He started off as my sponsor and we became friends. But first and foremost he is my sponsor.

So don't find yourself a pushover that you can manipulate. Make sure he or she has a solid recovery going before you ask. And make sure you ask! We need you as a leader, too!

Do you remember the last lie you told someone so they could help you to continue your downfall into addiction? Think for a moment. Was it a lie you told to manipulate someone to help you? It is hoped that your mind is a little more clear since the time you told that lie.

Think for another moment while putting yourself in the place of the person you lied to. Now, would you believe it if someone came to you with that same lie? Probably not. And they probably didn't either. We impugn or challenge our own integrity for the sake of our addiction, which lowers our self-worth to ourselves and to others.

Those people who you lied to probably tried at first to give you the benefit of the doubt, so as not to embarrass you or start a conflict.

The further you get into your recovery the more you'll see that the phrase "stinkin' thinkin' " applied to you in your addiction.

As addicts, we tend to rationalize and justify our actions and behaviors. As our mind clears up, we see how insane our thinking really was.

Do you feel a little embarrassed or ashamed? Good! I hope you do. Embarrassment lets you know that you do have a conscience. Having a conscience reminds you of the right and wrong you have done to yourself and others. With a conscience comes remorse, and we can try to make amends to ourselves and others.

The best way you can make amends to anyone is to get recovery and live it. Remember, actions speak louder than any words. You can tell someone you are trying in recovery, but showing them will leave a better impression.

If you tell someone something, they may remember. If you show someone, they will believe. But if you involve someone, they will understand.

So, involve the people you care about in your recovery. I'm talking about real friends and family. Not Pookie, Junebug, and Ray Ray.

You involved them involuntarily in your addiction. Now acknowledge you want their help in your recovery.

You are judged by the company you keep. Your mom and dad, or wife may not take your recovery seriously or believe you are really trying if they see you still running with your using buddies. They knew you had a problem when you were hanging with Pookie, Junebug, and Ray Ray. Then you claim to have recovery but they still see you hanging with the same crowd. Your credibility will go to the toilet. You have to shake off your using buddies and establish credibility.

The people who mean the most to you may not believe your sincerity in recovery at first. This will take time. Don't be discouraged or offended that you may be under a microscope with these people. Don't be angry that they don't trust like you think they should. Trust is to be earned, not given. Besides, you may have disappointed them, and letting down their guard may be difficult. Be patient; don't be in a hurry. Your recovery will show in your actions in time.

Your past use, and the damage done, could make this tough. But if you are in fact sincere, your family will trust and rebuild trust and faith in you once again.

I can remember one of my sponsees calling me and saying he used because everyone kept blaming or accusing him of using. "So," he said, "they keep blaming me for it, may as well do it."

I told him he was full of it. That was just an excuse for him to go use again. I told him all he did was remove any doubt that he wasn't done using out there in the streets. Do not let this sad, weak-minded excuse be yours.

You made the bed, so you lie in it. Take responsibility for the damage you've done to yourself and to others. Don't go giving yourself a poor-you pity-party. It's not gonna change the fact that your family may have lost confidence in you.

What will change that fact is ACTION. So take action against being an addict. Take your life seriously and your family will see your efforts in time. It may not be tomorrow or next week, but it will happen for sure. They need time to heal from the hurt you have caused them. If all this is worth it to you, you will be patient. Besides, it's your fault they lost this trust in you. You can't blame them for what you created.

Here's what I say about that… If you don't like something, change it. **If you can't change it, change your attitude!**

Alcoholics Anonymous lends its Big Book to Cocaine Anonymous, and they have agreed not to lend the name to any outside enterprise. The book you are now reading would be considered an outside enterprise. I cannot talk about what's in the Big Book except to say I highly recommend that you obtain one and work the Twelve Steps of the book. I advise you do this with a sponsor. Remember you can't do this alone, even if it is a selfish program!

To just say no and walk away sounds easy. But we are addicts. We can't just walk away—whatever your family or anyone who has not been there may think. We can't stop. How many times have you tried to quit using? How long did it last?

Control is an illusion; there is only one in control and that is God. You can't control anything. Not before, not today, not ever. You can, however, get a handle on addiction. This is not something that has to be in your life.

You may say you tried to control it, and not use. You didn't get control because you never had control. My advice is: **Let go and let God.** He will take control of what's going on in your life. You need to look at your willingness. You see he (God) gives us free will, or choice. As addicts we seem to make poor choices. Seek the guidance of your higher power and your support network.

Hang out with people in recovery. You will find, in time you have lots in common—more than you thought at first. The things you may find in recovery won't only be about recovery. With this important group of people, you will find and share remarkable coincidences and many of the same interests.

When you begin working the steps of recovery, you'll find that you already knew much of what you'll learn. It will be confirmation of what you already know. The difference is: **Working these steps will reconfirm what you need to do and ways to make it happen.**

Don't think you can't do it. **Think: How can I?** That's the difference between success and failure. That's not only the way to think for recovery, but life in general. Show faith in your higher power, keep in mind that faith without work is dead. Pray about it, but also work toward making the prayer materialize. My example to this is: If you pray for a job, you don't expect a job to come knocking on the door. You have to go look for a job. That's the work.

So again, faith without work is dead. Pray about it, and work on it, too.

I'm a firm believer that you become a product of your environment. If you hang around drugs and drug users, you become that. If you hang around recovery, you get recovery.

I also feel that negative brings on negative. Someone with a bad attitude often rubs off and gives others the same poor disposition.

As will positive bring positive results. Example: If you are broke and without a job, hang around someone who has a job. They may help you or give you ideas on attaining a job.

In order to make changes from one thing to move on to something better, you have to make some changes.

DARE TO DREAM, DARE TO LIVE THAT DREAM

WHAT WAS YOUR LIFE LIKE before drugs, and what do you dream it can be in recovery? If you can dream it, you can live it. You just have to find out how to make those dreams happen. What you dare to dream, dare to do. None of us dreamed as a child or as an adult that we wanted to be an addict. The reality is we don't have to be. I hear in recovery rooms all the time, the phrase "Fake it till you make it." This is a load of bull! Don't be fake about any aspect of your recovery. Approach it openly and honestly. Don't fake anything. If you have any problems or worries, that's why it's suggested you have a sponsor or a counselor to go to. This phrase "Fake it till you make it" contradicts the rigorous honesty that it really takes to obtain a clean and sober lifestyle. Nonetheless, you can make the change if you really want to. Something else really important: Do not straddle the proverbial fence. In other words: Don't put one foot in recovery and the other foot in the street with Pookie, Junebug, and Ray Ray. This will only prolong your addiction. Imagine that you literally are straddling a fence.

You have one leg on one side of the fence and one leg on the other. With a fence between your legs, what progress can you make doing anything? I don't see it possible to do anything productive. You stand there in a rut. That's exactly what it will be if you don't fully commit to recovery. So please make the conscious decision to get it right. In my recovery, I've found that the possibilities to do whatever I want to be successful are virtually limitless. The positive thinkers will succeed while negative thinkers will struggle in anything they do or attempt to do. There is power in positive thinking. Every day that you do not use, that is a positive thing. Every day is not going to be a good day. That's life. God promised us a good life, not a perfect one. Even though the day may not be a good day, it still can be a positive one by not using. Winners don't quit when they want to achieve. When life deals you a bad hand, you don't have to keep that hand. Re-deal the cards and play a whole new hand. Play the game you can win. No one wins in the dope game. Especially the users. Even the dealers' luck runs out eventually.

RELATIONSHIP AND RECOVERY

I AM NOT A PSYCHOLOGIST, but I do know it is not advisable to enter into a deeply personal relationship in the early stages of recovery. Get yourself together first, before adding the weight of such a relationship. Especially someone new to recovery. I have been to several inpatient treatment centers to facilitate meetings, and I see co-ed centers where they hold some of the meetings with both sexes. I see crushes and latching on to each other. Those relationships hardly ever work, and this hinders the recovery process. Imagine two people with twisted, addictive thinking and behaviors trying to hook up. You know they say, sick + sick = sicker. If you are already married, ask your spouse to please be patient with you. Without recovery you don't have much of a relationship with your spouse. So ask them to allow you to begin getting better before doing anything rash. If your spouse uses too, well, you have some major decisions to make. You know you have to stay away from using people if you want to have a real chance at recovery. I would suggest you both go to inpatient treatment—or at least one of you. I would hope both of you will want to make this change. In reality it doesn't always work out, but

I wish those of you with this dilemma the best of luck. In reference to your higher power, my higher power says to seek first the kingdom of God and his righteousness, and all things will be added to you. If you look at the situation from this perspective, if you don't look after yourself first, not only will no things be added to you, most certainly you will sacrifice many things. As they say, you cannot take care of anyone until you can take care of yourself. Just like you cannot make anyone happy unless you are happy yourself. Are you happy in your addiction? Then I really don't think you can make anyone else happy. Let me shoot very straight with you. Unless you make up your mind that you really want recovery, nothing that you read, see, or hear, is going to make a difference. The things that you read, see, or hear about recovery can and will help only if this is what you want. You will have to follow the advice of your counselors, sponsor, and people who already have what it is you're trying to get. There is absolutely no reason for them to steer you wrong. People who are forced into recovery rarely get it. Those who are made to go to treatment by the courts, or family… their chances of getting and keeping recovery are very slim. They are only getting clean to please the judge or that family member. If it's not from you, it's not going to last. Even though we as addicts need treatment, unless we surrender and go, somebody else forcing us in will just prolong or delay us coming to our own decision to get clean. You can be given the tools to use to get clean, but if you are not ready to use them, it won't do any good. Those tools will be useless to you. If you are given the tools to build a house but have no idea how to build a house, what kind of house can you build? If you are taught how to build a house and don't use the tools you were given to build that house, is your house gonna get built? Your recovery is going to work the same way. You can be given the tools and guidance to build recovery. If you don't follow this guidance or use the tools given, your results will be nil.

As the norm, two of the strongest muscles in our bodies are the mind (brain) and the heart. As drugs and alcohol take over, the very same muscles become the weakest. The mind is weakened by drugs and alcohol, which cloud the very judgment we would otherwise call good. It is so weakened by drugs and alcohol that we as addicts do the wrong thing and make the wrong decisions, knowing we are making a bad choice while making that very choice. It's been said by doctors that there is no physical addiction to cocaine or meth. It's been said that you can only be physically addicted to heroin and alcohol. This stands to reason that there are only methadone clinics and not cocaine clinics. This may also be the reason there is Antabuse for alcoholics and no pill or dose like methadone for cocaine or meth addicts. What doctors are saying is that our addiction is not physical, it's mental.

I argue that point with these questions:

- If this is not a physical addiction, why the weight loss, and softening of teeth and gums?

- Why can't you eat and sleep under the influence of these drugs?

- Why does meth make you pick at your skin?

We all know there are psychological effects, but the things I just described sure sound physical to me. By a doctor's standard, it is not a physical addiction, so that means one of the strongest muscles in our body becomes weak by our choosing to use these drugs. The heart becomes physically and emotionally weak. Do you know of any illegal substance that makes you healthy? With that alone in mind, no way is the heart any healthier by doing drugs. Emotionally we become crippled, or numb to our conscience, fearing being exposed as an addict.

We become liars. We will lie about even the smallest things, further damaging and enhancing the shame of our addiction. So, my point is: Two of the strongest muscles in our bodies are the two weakest as we use drugs.

OTHER NOT-SO-GOOD THINGS ABOUT ADDICTION

ASIDE FROM LOSING WEIGHT BY using cocaine or heroin, which in the streets they call the Jenny Crack diet, other physical effects are dilated eyes, which are a dead giveaway that you're under the influence of something. Then there's the sweat. Almost always, the body will perspire. That's because that crap comes out of your pores. Then if you have been away from the shower or bath for a day or two (known to happen a lot), you stink, and way worse than if you just played an intense game of ball. We tend to neglect these things because we can't seem to tear ourselves away from the dope long enough to take care of personal hygiene. For some odd reason—and I've asked several people about this—when we are high we don't often look in the mirror. I wonder, is this because we are tweakin and too busy peeking out doors and windows, or subconsciously we are ashamed of what we see in the mirror as a result of using? Maybe the fact is we are ashamed of what we have become.

And when we do look in the mirror, do we really see what others see? Are we afraid of looking in the mirror to further our denial? Maybe by looking, really looking at ourselves, we may see just how bad we have gotten. Nobody wants to really admit they fell off and have a problem with drugs. Those in denial don't feel they have a problem. They think the only problem they have is when they run out of drugs!

What is being shared is the common experience and the reality of this unpleasant experience. Also some solutions, ideas, and tools, if you will, to change things for the better. Some of what you have read here should serve as confirmation to what you already knew. And be something you can relate or connect to. By any means, I hope this is serving you as reality and confirmation that there is something better than being an addict. I have referred to myself on and off in this book. Much of what I have learned has been through my own experience with drugs and with recovery. I hated what I had become. My mother didn't teach me that drug stuff; I learned it all from Pookie, Junebug, and Ray Ray. I was not representing my mother or my family. I was shaming them and myself.

You must live life on life's terms. Sometimes it's very uncomfortable. There are many reasons people have to run from their lives. Where are you running to? When you self-medicate to hide from the reality of your life, it's only a temporary fix and in the reality of things it's not a fix at all. The problems will still be there when you sober up or come down from your high. And you may have made matters worse. Some of us have addictive personalities. We become equally addicted to the game. Even though it is not a game, it's called the dope game. We become addicted and get a rush from not only the drugs we use, but the whole process of the hunt, the score, the whole lifestyle of using.

That's why it's so important that if you want recovery, you have to change everything you do. Because many of us are addicted to the routine. Not using may be a good start but if you change nothing else, you are a relapse waiting to happen. You don't only have to clean your body but also your mind of the addictive behaviors. Some may find this a bit overwhelming. That's why it's so important to have a sponsor and work the suggested steps to recovery. I'll say this again: Nothing that's worth having is easy, or everyone would have it. Please don't allow complacency to jump into your recovery. Keep your guard up. Maintain level-headed thinking. Stay in constant contact with your sponsor or somebody who is clean and sober to help you stay that way. Don't be too proud to ask for help. Don't be too embarrassed to ask for help, either. You probably weren't too proud or embarrassed to ask for a front while in your addiction and your supply or money ran out. So don't be afraid to ask for help now that it's important. Maybe even life-and-death important. Sometimes, just having somebody say what you already know will help you stay on the right path. Just as you followed Pookie, Junebug, and Ray Ray down that destructive path… you must follow someone on the path to recovery. Remember, you must first follow in order to lead. Nobody owes you anything; not me, not your family, not the government, nobody. There are programs that can help. So don't let money, or lack thereof, be the reason you don't get help. Now's the time to make that very big step, to get your life back together.

Here are only a few things I will review with you, that are suggested to help you on your way.

- First, you have to make a conscious decision to seriously get clean and sober, and work a recovery program. Your best thinking had you snorting, shooting, and smoking.

- Second, you only have to change one thing! EVERYTHING! If you think there is a softer, easier way, you are in denial. You can't leave your life the way it is and just not use. It's not going to work.

- Third, find an inpatient or outpatient treatment, and learn what's needed to keep recovery.

- Fourth, go to meetings. It doesn't matter if it's CA, AA, or NA. Go to and be around people striving to stay clean.

- Fifth, find a sponsor and a support network. Keep his/her phone number handy, as well as a support network to help in tough moments.

Life gives you what you need to learn.

Use the following pages to write about or draw your own Positive Thoughts and Ideas, Looking Forward Dreams, To-Do List, Amends List, Promises, Personal Goals, and Achievements. In closing, I offer my most sincere good luck and prayers for you and your families. Please read this and any other literature that will help detour your addiction. Keep reading and you too can relate to recovery.

Positive Thoughts, Ideas

Positive Thoughts, Ideas

Positive Thoughts, Ideas

Positive Thoughts, Ideas

Looking Forward Dreams

Looking Forward Dreams

Looking Forward Dreams

Looking Forward Dreams

To-Do List

To-Do List

To-Do List

To-Do List

Amends List

Amends List

Amends List

Amends List

Promises

Promises

Promises

Promises

Personal Goals

Personal Goals

Personal Goals

Personal Goals

Achievements

Achievements

Achievements

Achievements

www.ingramcontent.com/pod-product-compliance
Lightning Source LLC
LaVergne TN
LVHW020430080526
838202LV00055B/5106